ESSENTIAL GUIDE TO ALOPECIA AREATA

Comprehensive Insights for Understanding, Managing, and Treating Hair Loss

DR. CASEY LOREN

DISCLAIMER

This book's content is only meant to be used for general informative purposes. Although the author has taken great care to ensure the content is accurate and thorough, no warranties or assurances on the information's accuracy, correctness, or reliability are provided. It is recommended that readers employ their own judgment and discretion when applying any material found in this book to their particular situation.

The information in this book is not intended to replace professional advice, nor is the author an expert in any of the subjects covered. It is recommended that readers consult with experienced professionals regarding any particular issues or concerns.

Any name that may be mentioned or referred in this book does not imply endorsement, recommendation, or relationship on the part of the author with any person, entity, good, website, or association. These references are made only for informational purposes and are not meant to be taken as recommendations or endorsements.

The information contained in this book may cause readers to suffer loss or damage, for which the author disclaims all obligation and accountability. The only people accountable for the decisions and actions taken by readers using the information presented are themselves.

Any names, characters, companies, locations, activities, occasions, and incidents referenced in this book are either made up or the result of the author's imagination. Any likeness to real people, living or dead, or to real things is entirely coincidental.

This book's content may change at any time, without prior notice, according to the author.

The onus is on the reader to verify whether there have been any updates or revisions.

The reader accepts the conditions of this disclaimer by reading this book. Please do not read this book or use its contents if you do not agree to these terms.

CHAPTER 1

KNOWLEDGE ABOUT ALOPECIA AREATA

Comprehensive Overview of Alopecia Areata

Alopecia Areata Overview

An autoimmune disease called alopecia areata is typified by abrupt, non-scarring hair loss. Although it can affect any part of the body that bears hair, it usually appears as oval or round patches of hair loss on the scalp. Men and women are both susceptible to the illness, which can strike at any age. Individual differences exist in the degree of hair loss and regeneration caused by Alopecia Areata.

Background and History

Ancient manuscripts have accounts of alopecia areata, which has been known for millennia. The word "alopecia" is derived from the Greek word "alopex," which means "fox," because the disease's hair loss is similar to fox mange. With major advancements in the 20th and 21st centuries concerning the autoimmune nature of Alopecia Areata and its genetic predispositions, medical understanding of the condition has changed over time.

Demographics and Epidemiology

Alopecia Areata affects about 2% of people worldwide. Although it can occur at any age, childhood or adolescence is usually when it initially manifests. Because there is no discernible gender tendency, it affects men and women in the same way. All racial and ethnic groups are affected, though the condition's prevalence may vary within some populations.

Alopecia Areata Types

Alopecia Areata is categorized into multiple kinds according to the type and severity of hair loss:

1. **Patchy Alopecia Areata**

- The most prevalent type, which is indicated by one or more oval or round patches of hair loss on the scalp or other parts of the body. If these patches combine, greater hair loss may result.

2. **Total Alopecia**

- A more severe variation in which all scalp hair is lost. Patients may continue to have hair in other body areas.

3. **Universal Alopecia**

- The most severe type, which causes total hair loss on the body and scalp, including facial hair, lashes, and eyebrows.

Signs and Cause of Death

Alopecia Areata symptoms generally consist of:

Abrupt hair loss in isolated areas.

- Hairs with an exclamation mark, which are short and taper at the root.

Itching or tingling in the afflicted regions.

The primary method of diagnosis is clinical, relying on the distinctive appearance of hair loss. Exclamation mark hairs are one example of a characteristic that dermoscopy can help identify. A scalp biopsy, which reveals peribulbar lymphocytic infiltration, a characteristic of the condition, helps confirm the diagnosis in cases when the diagnosis is unclear.

Genetic Elements

An important factor in Alopecia Areata is genetics. Strong risk factors include family history, and the disease has been linked to multiple genetic loci. These loci support the autoimmune theory of Alopecia Areata since they are frequently engaged in immune system control. The most well-known linked genes are those that belong to the complex known as HLA (human leukocyte antigen).

Triggers in the Environment

Genetically predisposed individuals may experience Alopecia Areata in response to environmental influences. Among these triggers are:

- Stress on the mind.

Infections caused by viruses.

- Trauma to the body.

Modifications in hormones.

Although these factors may hasten the onset of Alopecia Areata, research is still being done to determine the precise processes by which they do so.

Immune Processes

The main cause of alopecia areata is an autoimmune disorder in which hair follicles are accidentally attacked by the body's immune system, resulting in hair loss. Hair development is stopped when the immune system attacks anagen (active growth phase) hair follicles. T-lymphocytes—in particular, CD8+ T cells—are essential to this immunological reaction.

Psychological Effect

There can be significant psychological effects from Alopecia Areata. Hair loss can have an impact on one's overall quality of life, body image, and self-esteem. People who have alopecia areata may feel depressed, anxious, or emotionally distressed. Counseling and psychological support are crucial parts of managing the illness.

Typical Myths and Misunderstandings

There are various myths and misconceptions regarding Alopecia Areata, such as:

- **Myth:** Alopecia Areata is brought on by an infectious illness or inadequate hygiene.

Fact: It is not communicable and is an autoimmune illness unrelated to cleanliness.

- **Myth:** Alopecia Areata causes permanent hair loss.

Fact: There is a chance for hair regrowth, and the condition can fluctuate between periods of hair loss and regrowth.

Myth: Scalp is the only area affected by alopecia areata.

Fact: Any bodily part that bears hair may be affected.

For patients and their families to manage expectations and seek the right care and support, it is imperative that they are aware of these facts.

CHAPTER 2

REASONS AND DANGER ELEMENTS

Synopsis of Causes

An autoimmune condition called alopecia areata is typified by erratic, non-scarring hair loss on the scalp and other areas of the body. Although the exact origin of alopecia areata is unknown, a number of genetic, environmental, and immunological variables are thought to be involved. Hair loss results from the immune system attacking hair follicles inadvertently. Any age, gender, or ethnicity can be affected by this disorder, albeit some circumstances can increase its severity and onset.

Hereditary Propensity

In alopecia areata, **Genetic Predisposition** is a major factor. Studies show that alopecia areata and other autoimmune illnesses run in families, increasing the risk of getting the condition in affected individuals. Alopecia areata has been connected to multiple genes related to immune system control, indicating a possible genetic component. Alopecia areata patients frequently have certain genetic markers, such as those in the HLA (human leukocyte antigen) region, which lends credence to the idea that genetic factors influence vulnerability.

Immune System Impairment

Since **Immune System Dysfunction** is a major contributing factor to the development of alopecia areata, the condition is essentially an autoimmune one. Under this syndrome, hair follicles are mistakenly targeted by the immune system, which believes they are foreign invaders. Hair loss is the result of this immune attack's inflammation and disruption of the function of the hair follicles. T cells, in particular CD8+ cytotoxic T lymphocytes, are important participants in this immune response because they invade hair follicles and cause their death.

Emotional and Stressful Elements

Alopecia areata is known to worsen in response to **Stress and Emotional Factors**. Although stress by itself is unlikely to be the cause of the disorder, in vulnerable individuals it may initiate or exacerbate hair loss. Stress on an emotional level can alter the body physiologically by increasing the production of stress hormones like cortisol, which can affect inflammation and the immune system. Patients frequently report periods of hair loss that come after major life stressors, suggesting a strong link between emotional health and alopecia areata expression.

Effects of Hormones

Compared to other factors, the involvement of **Hormonal Influences** in alopecia areata is less obvious. Hormones are thought to affect the immune system and the cycling of hair follicles, though. Hormonal changes that occur during puberty, pregnancy, or menopause may have an impact on the onset or course of alopecia areata. Furthermore, this disorder is frequently linked to thyroid disease, which entails hormonal imbalances, underscoring the possibility that hormones play a role in alopecia areata.

Dietary Inadequacies

Nutritional Deficiencies may contribute to alopecia areata and have an effect on the general health of hair. Conditions causing hair loss have been linked to deficiencies in specific vitamins and minerals, including zinc, iron, vitamin D, and biotin. These nutrients are necessary to boost the immune system and keep hair follicles in good condition. Although alopecia areata is unlikely to be caused by nutritional deficiencies alone, they can make the condition worse or prevent hair from growing back.

Diseases and Infections

There are some **Infections and Illnesses** that can cause or exacerbate alopecia areata. Viruses such as the CMV or Epstein-Barr virus have been linked to the development of autoimmune diseases, such as alopecia areata. Alopecia areata patients frequently have other immune system-compromising conditions including vitiligo, lupus, or autoimmune thyroid disease, which raises the possibility of a connection between systemic health issues and hair loss.

Drugs and Medical Procedures

Alopecia areata is one condition that can occasionally be brought on by **Medications and Treatments**. Some medications, such as those used in chemotherapy, can cause hair loss by interfering with cells that divide quickly, such as hair follicles. In those who are predisposed, other immune-suppressive drugs such as biologics or interferons may also cause alopecia areata. When addressing alopecia areata, it's critical for patients and healthcare professionals to take into account any possible pharmaceutical adverse effects.

Exposures to the Environment

Alopecia areata may develop as a result of **Environmental Exposures**. Pollution, pollutants, and allergens are a few examples of factors that can affect immune function and perhaps set off autoimmune reactions. Furthermore, alterations in weather patterns or exposure to ultraviolet radiation can have an effect on the health of skin and hair, potentially aggravating alopecia areata in vulnerable individuals.

Considerations for Age, Gender, and Ethnicity

Understanding alopecia areata requires taking **Age, Gender, and Ethnicity Considerations** into account. Though it can affect anyone at any age, children and young people are the ones who are diagnosed with it most frequently. Both sexes are impacted, yet some research indicates that the frequency and severity of the condition fluctuate slightly depending on gender. Another factor is ethnicity, as different ethnic groups have differing rates and presentations of alopecia areata. It is possible to improve patient care and treatment approaches by having a better understanding of these demographic characteristics.

CHAPTER 3

Identification and Medical Assessment

Essential Guide to Alopecia Areata: Medical Evaluation and Diagnosis

The autoimmune condition known as alopecia areata is typified by the abrupt start of patchy hair loss on the scalp and other body areas. For management and treatment to be successful, a proper diagnosis and medical evaluation are essential. An in-depth summary of the most important factors in the diagnosis and assessment of alopecia areata is given in this guide.

First Appointment and Medical History

Significance

The diagnosis of alopecia areata relies heavily on the initial visit and a comprehensive patient history. Knowing the patient's medical, family, and lifestyle history can help rule out other possible reasons for hair loss and offer important hints.

Important Elements

1. **Health History**:

- Past medical issues, particularly those related to the autoimmune system (e.g., diabetes, thyroid illness).

- A history of skin disorders or allergies.

- Hair loss experiences in the past and their results.

2. **History of the Family**:

- Any family members suffering from autoimmune diseases such as alopecia areata.

- Genetic inheritance patterns and predispositions.

3. **Environmental and Lifestyle Factors**:

Stress levels as well as recent traumatic experiences.

- Nutritional status and eating patterns.

- Toxin or chemical exposure.

4. **Drugs and Medical Interventions**:

- Prescription and over-the-counter medications, as well as vitamins.

The efficaciousness of earlier hair loss treatments.

Consultation with the Patient

Getting detailed information can be aided by conducting an organized interview with open-ended questions. Building a relationship with the patient is crucial in order to promote transparency and candor.

Physical Inspection

Goal

During the physical examination, the patient's general health is evaluated, and any symptoms that could point to alopecia areata or other underlying disorders are looked for.

Examining Procedures

1. **Physical Examination in General**:

Evaluate the patient's overall look and nutritional condition.

- Look for indications of systemic illnesses, such as nail pitting and vitiligo.

2. **Evaluation of Scalp**:

Examine the scalp to determine the degree and patterns of hair loss.

- Keep an eye out for indications of inflammation, scarring, or other skin disorders.

3. **Examination of Nails**:

- Check nails for alopecia areata-related anomalies such as pitting, ridging, or other irregularities.

Examination of the Hair and Scalp

To differentiate alopecia areata from other forms of hair loss, alopecia areata characteristics must be carefully observed on the scalp and hair.

1. **Examining Visually**:

- Determine the location and amount of hair loss.

- Look for any hairs with an exclamation mark, which are broken hairs that are shorter at the root.

2. **Hair Pull Test**:

- To determine the fragility and loss rate of hair, gently tug on a small section of hair.

- Active hair loss may be indicated by a positive pull test result (more than 5–10 hairs).

Alopecia Areata Dermoscopy

Position

Alopecia areata can be diagnosed with the use of dermoscopy, a non-invasive diagnostic technique that improves the visibility of hair and scalp features.

Features of the Dermis
1. **Pink Circles**:

- Show keratin and sebum-filled follicular ostia.

2. **Dark Circles**:

- Stand in for fractured hair shafts inside of follicles.

3. **Hairs with exclamation marks**:

- Short, broken hairs that taper down to the scalp.

4. **Hairs of Vellus**:

- Short, thin hairs that point to hair regeneration.

Benefits
- Increases the accuracy of diagnosis.

- Makes it possible to identify small changes early.

Tracks the effectiveness of treatment over time.

Laboratory Work and Blood Testing

Goal
Laboratory testing assists in ruling out alternative diagnoses and identifying underlying causes or related disorders.

Typical Exams

1. **CBC, or complete blood count**:

Evaluate general well-being and detect infections or anemia.

2. **Tests for Thyroid Function**:

- Look for thyroid conditions that are frequently linked to alopecia areata.

3. **Screening for Autoantibodies**:

- Recognises autoimmune diseases (ANA, rheumatoid factor, etc.).

4. **Studies on Iron**:

- Exams for iron deficiency, as this condition may aggravate hair loss.

5. **Levels of Vitamin D**:

Examines for deficiencies that might affect the regulation of the immune system.

Skin Biopsy

Indication

When the diagnosis is unclear or in order to rule out other disorders, a skin biopsy is carried out.

Method

1. **Anaesthesia Local**:

- To reduce discomfort, numb the biopsy site.

2. **Punch Biopsy**:

- For histological analysis, a little, circular piece of skin, usually 4 mm in diameter, is removed.

3. **Examination of Histopathology**:

- Recognises distinctive characteristics such as preserved sebaceous glands, miniaturized hair follicles, and peribulbar lymphocytic infiltrates, or "swarm of bees."

Advantages

Verifies the alopecia areata diagnosis.

- Sets apart from other alopecias that leave scars and others that do not.

Contrastive Diagnosis

Significance

Making the distinction between alopecia areata and other hair loss conditions guarantees that the right care and therapy are provided.

Common Diagnoses Made by Differential

1. **Alopecia Androgenetic**:

- Gradual thinning and patterning of hair loss, usually excluding the frontal hairline in women.

2. **Effluvium Telogen**:

- Uniform hair thinning and diffuse loss in the wake of stress or sickness.

3. **Tinea Capitis**:

- Fungal infection of the scalp, which frequently manifests as hair breakage and scaling.

4. **Redneck mania**:

- Hair loss from obsessive hair tugging; frequently, this results in uneven areas with different hair lengths.

5. **Planopilaris Lizchen**:

- An inflammatory disorder of the scalp that results in permanent hair loss and scars.

Psychological Evaluation

Importance

Significant psychological effects of alopecia areata might include despair, anxiety, and low self-esteem.

Elements of the Assessment

1. **Psychological Assessment**:

Evaluate the patient's emotional and psychological health.

- Check for mental health conditions such as depression, anxiety, and others.

2. **Measurement of Life Quality**:

- Assess how hair loss affects everyday activities and social relationships.

Assistance and Steps

Therapy and support networks.

- Making referrals to mental health specialists when necessary.

- Stress reduction strategies.

Dermatologists' Role

Proficiency

Dermatologists are experts in identifying and treating disorders of the skin and hair, such as alopecia areata.

1. **Diagnosis**:

- Perform comprehensive dermoscopic and clinical evaluations.

- Place and interpret the required biopsies and laboratory testing.

2. **Planning for Treatment**:

- Create customized treatment programs depending on the degree and type of hair loss.

- Provide medical care, including systemic medicines, immunotherapy, and topical corticosteroids.

3. **Observation**:

- Frequent check-ins to evaluate therapy response and modify remedies as necessary.

4. **Education of Patients**:

- Inform patients about the illness, available treatments, and techniques for taking care of themselves.

Additional Expert Consultations

Multidisciplinary Method

For thorough management, it could occasionally be required to confer with external experts.

Possible Experts

1. **Endocrine specialists**:

- Take care of related endocrine conditions, like thyroid issues.

2. **Patheumatologists**:

- Take care of any autoimmune diseases that alopecia areata may coexist with.

3. **Psychiatrists and psychologists**:

- Offer mental health assistance to individuals coping with the psychological effects of hair loss.

4. **Dietitians**:

- Offer food advice and supplement recommendations to promote general health and hair development.

Cooperation

A comprehensive approach to patient care, covering both the physical and psychological components of alopecia areata, is ensured by effective communication and collaboration among professionals.

In conclusion, a multidisciplinary team for holistic care, a complete patient history, a physical examination, and sophisticated diagnostic technologies like dermoscopy are all important components of a comprehensive approach to the diagnosis and medical evaluation of alopecia areata. The quality of life and results for patients can be greatly enhanced by appropriate diagnosis and customized treatment programs.

CHAPTER 4

CONVENTIONAL THERAPY CHOICES

Comprehensive Guide to Alopecia Areata: Conventional Therapy Approaches

An autoimmune disease called alopecia areata is typified by patchy hair loss on the scalp and other body areas. Even though the precise etiology of the problem is still unknown, a number of conventional therapy options are available to help manage it and encourage hair growth. To assist patients and healthcare professionals in making educated decisions, this book offers a thorough summary of every available treatment option.

Corticosteroids Topical

Explanation:

Anti-inflammatory drugs called topical corticosteroids are administered topically to the afflicted area of the skin in order to lower inflammation and inhibit the immune system. They come in a variety of forms, such as lotions, ointments, gels, and creams.

Apply:

- Used on the bald areas once or twice a day.

- Fluocinonide, betamethasone dipropionate, and clobetasol propionate are examples of commonly used corticosteroids.

Achievement:

- Frequently beneficial for people with mild to moderate alopecia areata, including youngsters.

It can take a few weeks for the results to show.

Atrophy (thinning of the skin)

- Striae, or stretch marks

- Spider veins, or telangiectasia

- Systemic absorption that could result in adrenal suppression if used over an extended period of time.

Intralesional Injections of Steroids

Explanation:
In order to lessen inflammation and promote hair development, corticosteroids are injected directly into the bald areas during intralesional steroid injections.

Apply:
Usually given out by a dermatologist.

Triamcinolone acetonide is a corticosteroid that is frequently used.

- Every 4–6 weeks, injections are administered.

Achievement:
- Extremely successful in treating small, isolated alopecia areata spots.

- A few weeks following therapy, hair regrowth is visible.

Inverse Repercussions:
- Soreness or pain at the injection site.

- Atrophic skin.

- A hypo- or depigmented area where the injection was made.

Corticosteroids in the System

Explanation:

Oral or injectable drugs called systemic corticosteroids lower inflammation and weaken the immune system all over the body.

Apply:

- Frequently used in situations of alopecia areata that are severe or advancing quickly.

Prednisone and prednisolone are common drugs.

Achievement:

- Has the potential to stimulate hair growth, although the benefits could not persist long after stopping.

Because of the possible adverse effects, this medication is often only used temporarily.

Inverse Repercussions:
Gaining weight.

- Hypertension, or elevated blood pressure.

- Osteoporosis.

- An elevated infection risk.

- Variations in mood and psychological impacts.

Rogaine (minoxidil)

Explanation:
An over-the-counter topical medication called minoxidil stimulates hair follicles and encourages hair growth. It can be purchased as foam or in solutions of 2% and 5%.

Apply:
- Used on the scalp twice a day.

Appropriate for both genders.

Achievement:
Facilitates the extension of the hair follicles' growth phase.

- It could take three to six months to see results.

Dryness or inflammation of the scalp.

- The development of unwanted facial hair if the solution runs down the face.

- A little hair loss during the course of the first course of treatment.

Dritho-Scalp, or anthralin

Explanation:

Anthralin is a tar-like synthetic drug used to treat alopecia areata and psoriasis. It encourages hair growth and regulates the immunological system.

Apply:

- Used briefly (20–60 minutes) on the scalp before being removed with a wash (short-contact therapy).

- Usually used once every day.

Achievement:
- Works well for certain people, especially those with less severe alopecia areata.

- It can take several months before the results are apparent.

Inverse Repercussions:
- Skin irritation.

- Skin and hair discolorations that are transient.

- Contact dermatitis risk.

DPCP, or diphencyprone

Explanation:
A topical immunotherapy drug called diphencyprone causes a slight allergic reaction in order to boost the immune system and encourage the growth of hair.

Apply:
- First applied to cause sensitization by a dermatologist.

- Weekly applications of progressively higher concentrations come next.

Achievement:

- In those with severe alopecia areata, it may be beneficial.

It could take several months for hair to regrow.

Inverse Repercussions:

- Intense irritation from contact.

- Itching and blistering.

- Excessive or inadequate pigmentation.

SADBE, or squaric acid dibutyl ester

Explanation:

Similar to DPCP, SADBE is another topical immunotherapy drug that is intended to cause a minor allergic reaction and promote hair growth.

Apply

Weekly applications are made after the sensitization period.

Over time, concentration grew more and more focused.

Achievement:

Like DPCP, it can work well in long-term situations.

- After a few months, there was noticeable hair growth.

Inverse Repercussions:

- Dermatitis from contact.

- Itching and blistering.

Discoloration of the skin.

Immunotherapy

Explanation

Topical immunotherapy is the use of drugs such as SADBE or DPCP to change the immune system's activity and trigger an allergic response.

Apply:

- Under the direction and supervision of a dermatologist.

- Consistent administration, with dose modifications according to patient response.

Achievement:

- May be beneficial for severe or chronic alopecia areata sufferers.

It could take many months for hair regrowth to become apparent.

Inverse Repercussions:

Localized responses on the skin.

- Possibility of systemic allergic responses.

Discoloration of the skin.

Phototherapy

Explanation:

In order to reduce inflammation and promote hair growth, phototherapy, commonly referred to as light therapy, involves exposing the afflicted skin to ultraviolet (UV) light.

Apply:

- Applying UVB or UVA light in a therapeutic context; occasionally, this is coupled with a photosensitizing drug such as psoralen (PUVA therapy).

- Meetings held two or three times every week on average.

Achievement

- Varying outcomes; whereas some people may not respond, others may see notable regrowth.

- Long-term advantages lack solid evidence.

Burns on the skin.

- Long-term use increases the risk of skin cancer.

Early aging of the skin.

Benefits and Adverse Reactions

Changes dramatically depending on the patient and the kind of treatment.

- Success rates for immunotherapy drugs, minoxidil, and topical and intralesional corticosteroids vary.

- Combination treatments frequently produce superior outcomes.

Vary in severity from minor (dryness, irritation of the skin) to serious (corticosteroid systemic effects, increased risk of skin cancer from phototherapy).

- The significance of weighing potential negative effects against efficacy.

- Consistent monitoring and protocol adjustments for treatment to reduce adverse effects.

To sum up, conventional therapies for alopecia areata provide a variety of choices based on the intensity and scope of the illness. In order to choose the best course of therapy, patients and their healthcare providers should consult closely and weigh the advantages and disadvantages of each option. For the purpose of managing side effects and maximizing results, routine follow-up visits and treatment regimen modifications are essential.

CHAPTER 5

INNOVATIVE AND CUTTING-EDGE THERAPIES

Essential Guide to Advanced and Emerging Treatments for Alopecia Areata

An autoimmune disease called alopecia areata is typified by patchy hair loss. Although the precise cause is yet unknown, hair follicles are attacked by the immune system. In order to give patients and healthcare professionals a thorough knowledge, this book covers both cutting-edge and novel therapies for alopecia areata.

Inhibitors of Janus Kinase (JAK)

Synopsis

A class of drugs known as JAK inhibitors targets the Janus kinase enzyme family. These enzymes are essential to the signaling pathways of the immune system. JAK inhibitors can modify the immune response and lessen the autoimmune attack on hair follicles by blocking these enzymes.

Mode of Action

JAK inhibitors function by preventing one or more members of the Janus kinase family from acting (JAK1, JAK2, JAK3, and TYK2). This inhibition stops pro-inflammatory cytokines from signaling, which in turn stops the autoimmune attack on hair follicles.

Safety and Effectiveness

JAK inhibitors, such as tofacitinib and ruxolitinib, have demonstrated encouraging outcomes in clinical trials when it comes to encouraging hair regeneration in alopecia areata patients. Data on long-term safety and efficacy are still being gathered, though. An elevated risk of infections and possible abnormalities in liver enzymes are common side effects.

 Present Utilisation

Currently, alopecia areata is treated off-label with JAK inhibitors. Scholars persist in investigating their possibilities and want to obtain official authorization for this sign.

Treatment with Platelet-Rich Plasma (PRP)

Synopsis

To encourage hair growth, PRP therapy uses a concentrated sample of the patient's own blood platelets. Growth factors found in large quantities in platelets have the ability to activate hair follicles.

Method

1. **Blood Collection**: The patient has a tiny volume of blood taken.

2. **Centrifugation**: To separate the platelet-rich plasma from other blood components, the blood sample is spun in a centrifuge.

3. **Injection**: Alopecia areata-affected scalp regions receive an injection of PRP.

Safety and Effectiveness

Numerous patients have reported increased hair thickness and density following PRP treatment, which has produced encouraging outcomes in small-scale trials. Because the treatment is autologous, side effects are usually mild, though they can include mild bleeding and transient injection site soreness.

Present Utilisation

PRP is frequently utilized as a cosmetic treatment for hair loss, and as data demonstrating its effectiveness mounts, so does its application for alopecia areata.

Biologic Substances

Synopsis

Biologics are sophisticated medications that target particular immune system components and are derived from living organisms. They provide a focused method of treating autoimmune diseases, including alopecia areata.

Illustrations and Action Mechanism

- **Dupilumab**: Reduces inflammation by focusing on the interleukin-4 receptor.

- **Secukinumab**: This medication inhibits the cytokine interleukin-17, which is involved in inflammation.

Safety and Effectiveness

In addition to their proven efficacy in treating autoimmune illnesses in general, biologics may also be useful in treating alopecia areata, according to recent research. In addition to being costly, some medications may have major adverse effects, such as an increased risk of infection.

Present Utilisation

Biologics are approved to treat rheumatoid arthritis and psoriasis, but their application to alopecia areata is now mostly exploratory, awaiting larger-scale clinical trials.

Laser Therapy at Low Levels (LT)

Synopsis

Red or near-infrared light is used in LLLT to promote hair growth. The idea behind this non-invasive procedure is that light radiation can stimulate cell activity.

Mode of Action

LT is thought to:

- Boost the blood supply to the hair follicles.

- Promote protein synthesis and cellular metabolism.

Lessen the swelling that surrounds hair follicles.

Safety and Effectiveness

LLLT has been demonstrated in numerous trials to increase hair thickness and density. The primary side effect, slight scalp irritation, is regarded as normal.

Present Utilisation

Both clinical settings and at-home use are possible with LTE devices. They are starting to gain popularity as a non-invasive therapeutic option for patients.

Methods of Hair Transplantation

Synopsis

Hair follicles from one area of the body—usually the back of the scalp—are transplanted to the sections of the body affected by alopecia areata.

Methods

1. **Follicular Unit Transplantation (FUT)**: This procedure splits a scalp skin strip into individual follicular units, which are then transplanted.

2. **Follicular Unit Extraction (FUE)**: This method entails taking individual hair follicles

out of the donor region and depositing them elsewhere.

Safety and Effectiveness

Hair transplantation can increase hair density and produce long-lasting effects. However, because alopecia areata is an unexpected disorder, its efficacy may be limited. Infection and scarring are examples of complications.

Present Utilisation

While patients with stable alopecia areata and adequate donor hair may be candidates for hair transplantation, the procedure is mainly used for androgenetic alopecia.

Stem Cell Utilisation

Synopsis

Using stem cells, stem cell treatment aims to rejuvenate and repair damaged tissues, such as hair follicles.

Mode of Action

Because stem cells can develop into multiple cell types, they can help hair follicles regenerate and may even be able to stop an autoimmune onslaught.

Safety and Effectiveness

Stem cell therapy appears to be a potentially effective treatment for alopecia areata, according to preliminary research. While safety is still being assessed, immunological responses and tumor development are possible hazards.

Present Utilisation

Clinical trials are being conducted to ascertain the safety and efficacy of stem cell therapy for alopecia areata, which is currently in the experimental stage.

Immunomodulatory Substances

Synopsis

Drugs known as immunomodulators alter the immune system with the goal of lessening the autoimmune assault on hair follicles.

Instances

- **Methotrexate**: An immunosuppressive medication that is useful in extreme circumstances.

- **Cyclosporine**: An additional strong immunosuppressant that may help with alopecia areata.

Safety and Effectiveness

Immunomodulators have serious adverse effects, such as a heightened risk of infections, liver damage, and other systemic consequences, despite their potential benefits.

Present Utilisation

These medications are usually administered under strict medical supervision and saved for severe, unresponsive cases of alopecia areata.

Novel Topical Remedies

Synopsis

In order to deliver localized therapy with fewer systemic side effects, new topical therapies are being developed.

Instances

- **Topical JAK inhibitors**: Purport to offer the advantages of JAK inhibition without putting the body at risk.

- **Topical corticosteroids**: Keep improving them for increased safety and effectiveness.

Safety and Effectiveness

Early trials on novel topical therapies are encouraging, as new formulations strive to maximize efficacy and penetration while reducing adverse effects such as skin atrophy.

Present Utilisation

Some of these medications are already accessible for off-label usage, while others are undergoing various phases of clinical studies and research.

Combination Treatments

Synopsis

Combining various therapeutic approaches can improve results and address various alopecia areata pathways.

Instances

- **PRP in combination with microneedling**: Improves PRP efficacy and delivery.

- **JAK inhibitor and topical corticosteroid combination**: Seek to enhance each other's effects for improved results.

Safety and Effectiveness

Clinical trials are beginning to show promise for combination medicines, which may provide better outcomes with tolerable side effects. However in order to evaluate interactions and cumulative side effects, close observation is needed.

Present Utilisation

There is potential for more successful management of alopecia areata since combination medicines are being investigated more and more in clinical practice and research settings.

Clinical Trials and Advances in Research

Synopsis

Research and ongoing clinical studies are essential to improving our knowledge of alopecia areata and its management.

Presently Prioritised Areas

Genetic research: Determining the genetic components of alopecia areata.

- **Research on the immune system**: Determining the exact mechanisms underlying an autoimmune attack.

New treatments: Assessing the safety and effectiveness of cutting-edge medicines, such as stem cell therapy, biologics, and newly developed topical medications.

Significance

Important information from clinical trials is used to create novel treatments and influence treatment recommendations. Patients who take part in clinical trials may have access to innovative therapies.

Present Utilisation

Clinical trial participation is recommended in order to support ongoing research and maybe gain access to novel therapies. Medical professionals can assist patients in locating and signing up for suitable studies.

Final Thoughts

Alopecia areata is a complicated disorder for which there are a number of novel treatments that provide hope. The field of treating alopecia areata is quickly changing, ranging from stem cell therapy to JAK inhibitors. To make the best treatment decisions, patients and healthcare professionals should remain up to date on the most recent developments.

CHAPTER 6

ALTERNATIVE AND COMPLEMENTARY MEDICINE

Comprehensive Guide to Alternative and Complementary Therapies for Alopecia Areata

Diet and Nutritional Supplements

Overview

Hair loss is a symptom of the autoimmune disease alopecia areata. Diet and nutritional supplements can promote general health and possibly modulate immunological function, which might be important in controlling the illness.

Important Elements

1. **Biotin**: An important B vitamin for healthy hair. A lack of biotin may cause hair loss.

2. **Vitamin D**: Autoimmune diseases are associated with deficiencies. The immune system can be modulated with the aid of supplements.

3. **Zinc**: Essential for a healthy immune system and healthy hair growth. Hair loss is linked to low levels.

4. **Iron**: A common cause of hair loss, particularly in women, is iron deficiency anemia.

5. **Omega-3 Fatty Acids**: May lessen autoimmune activity due to its anti-inflammatory qualities.

Dietary Points to Remember

1. **Anti-inflammatory Diet**: Give special attention to foods like fruits, vegetables, whole grains, lean meats, and healthy fats that help to lower inflammation.

2. **Avoiding Allergens**: Food allergies might aggravate autoimmune reactions in certain people. Dairy products, gluten, and processed foods are frequently to blame.

3. **Hydration**: Enough water consumption is necessary for nutrient transport and general wellness.

Herbal Treatments

Well-Known Herbs

1. **Aloe Vera**: Well-known for its calming effects, aloe vera can be administered topically to lessen irritation and encourage the development of hair.

2.   **Ginseng**:   Supposed   to   promote circulation and lessen oxidative stress in order to promote hair development.

3. **Rosemary Oil**: To promote blood flow and stimulate hair follicles, rosemary oil is frequently applied topically.

4. **Saw palmetto**: This may inhibit the hormone that causes hair loss; especially useful in androgenetic alopecia but also maybe helpful in alopecia areata.

5. **Green Tea Extract**: This extract contains anti-inflammatory polyphenols.

Application and Setting Up

- **Topical Applications**: Numerous herbal medicines can be used directly on the scalp as DIY masks or as oils.

Oral Supplements: These come in the shape of tea or capsules. Dosage should be chosen after consulting a specialist and taking into account individual demands.

Chinese medicine

Idea

In order to encourage healing and enhance energy flow, acupuncture includes the insertion of tiny needles into particular bodily locations.

Advantages

1. **Boosts Blood Circulation**: Optimises the transport of nutrients to hair follicles.

2. **Decreases Stress**: Aids in regulating stress-related hormones, which may influence hair loss.

3. **Changes Immune Response**: Has the ability to change how the immune system targets hair follicles.

Method

- **Sessions**: Usually lasting 30 to 60 minutes, these sessions may be necessary once or twice a week for a few months.

Experience: Painless in most cases, emphasizing relaxation and general well-being.

Aromatherapy

Hair Growth Essential Oils

1. **Lavender**: Besides its sedative qualities, lavender helps stimulate hair growth.

2. **Peppermint**: Vitalizes the scalp and increases blood flow.

3. **Thyme**: Promotes a healthy scalp and possesses antibacterial qualities.

4. **Cedarwood**: Promotes better hair growth and oil-producing gland balance.

Methods of Application

- **Scalp Massage**: Apply a few drops of essential oil to your scalp after combining it with a carrier oil (such as coconut or jojoba).

- **Diffusion**: Setting up an essential oil diffuser can help create a relaxing atmosphere and lessen tension.

Hypnotherapy

Mechanism

Through focused attention and guided relaxation, hypnosis can raise one's level of awareness, which can reduce stress and change unfavorable thought patterns.

Alopecia Areata Benefits

Stress Reduction: Aids in the management of stress, which has been known to cause hair loss.

Changes in Behaviour: Promotes optimistic thinking and self-worth, which may have an effect on general health.

Procedure

Sessions: 45–60 minutes, usually; led by a certified hypnotherapist.

- **Experience**: Patients concentrate on relaxation and constructive recommendations while staying alert and in control.

Therapeutic Massage

Advantages

1. **Improves Circulation**: Promotes nutrient delivery by improving blood flow to the scalp.

2. **Reduces Stress**: Relieves strain and stress, both of which are known to be factors in hair loss.

3. **Stimulates Hair Follicles**: Growth can be enhanced by directly stimulating hair follicles.

Methods
- **Scalp Massage**: Uses light circular strokes to concentrate on the scalp.

- **Full Body Massage**: Enhances circulation throughout the body and lowers general stress.

Stress Reduction Methods

Significance

Alopecia areata is one of the autoimmune diseases that is known to be triggered by stress. Good stress management can reduce flare-ups and improve general well-being.

Methods

1. **Mindfulness Meditation**: Promotes mental clarity and calmness.

2. **Yoga**: Reduces stress by combining physical postures with breathing techniques.

3. **Inhalation Exercises**: Easy methods such as deep breathing can effectively lower stress levels.

Mental-Physical Therapies

Overview

Mind-body therapies promote holistic well-being by highlighting the relationship between mental and physical health.

Methods

1. **Meditation**: Promotes mental clarity and lowers stress.

2. **Tai Chi**: Enhances general health through thoughtful movements combined with gentleness.

3. **Biofeedback**: Reduces stress by teaching physiological regulation skills.

All-encompassing Methods

Philosophical

Restoring balance and encouraging spontaneous healing are the goals of holistic therapies, which take into account the full individual, including physical, emotional, and spiritual health.

Crucial Procedures

1.   **Integrated Medicine**: Blends complementary and alternative medicine.

2. **Naturopathy**: Promotes the body's natural healing process through lifestyle modifications and natural therapies.

3. **Functional Medicine** aims to locate and treat the underlying causes of illness.

Assessing Safety and Efficacy

Scientific Proof

- **Clinical Studies**: Assess alternative medicines' efficacy in controlled environments.

Patient Testimonials: First-hand accounts from individuals who have utilized these treatments.

Safety Points to Remember

Consult Healthcare Providers: Prior to beginning any new treatment, make sure you speak with a healthcare professional.

Supplement Quality: To prevent contamination and guarantee efficacy, be sure that your vitamins and herbs come from reliable suppliers.

- **Potential Interactions**: Be mindful of any possible conflicts with prescription drugs.

Different techniques of controlling alopecia areata are provided by complementary and alternative therapies. These therapies can assist hair regrowth and complement traditional treatments since they provide an emphasis on general health and well-being. But it's critical to assess each therapy's safety and effectiveness, ideally with medical professionals' help.

CHAPTER 7

ADAPTATION AND PSYCHOLOGICAL ASSISTANCE

Alopecia Areata Essential Guide: Managing and Seeking Psychological Assistance

An autoimmune condition called alopecia areata is typified by abrupt hair loss, frequently in circular regions. Alopecia Areata can have significant psychological and emotional effects in addition to its physical ones. This manual offers a thorough summary of coping techniques and sources of support to assist people in addressing the psychological and emotional difficulties linked to this illness.

Hair Loss's Emotional Effects

A wide range of emotions, such as astonishment, sadness, anger, and grief, can be brought on by abrupt hair loss. It's critical to understand that these emotions are typical. Losing hair can have an impact on social relationships and self-esteem because hair is frequently intimately associated with identity and self-image. People could encounter:

- **Depression and Anxiety**: Feelings of depression and anxiety may be brought on by or made worse by hair loss. It's normal to feel out of control and to worry about how other people will see you.

- **Grief and Mourning**: Losing hair can cause one to feel as though a piece of themselves has been taken away. The grieving process after this and other major losses is comparable.

- **Social Isolation**: Withdrawing from social interactions out of a fear of stigmatization or judgment can leave some people feeling alone and lonely.

Coping Mechanisms and Strategies

Creating efficient coping mechanisms is essential to controlling the psychological effects of Alopecia Areata. Among these tactics are:

- **Acknowledgment and Acceptance**: The first step in learning to cope with hair loss is to acknowledge and accept your feelings.

Education and Information: Reducing feelings of isolation can be accomplished by being aware of the condition and the fact that anyone can be affected by it, regardless of age, gender, or background.

- **Creative Expression**: Writing, drawing, or creating music are examples of creative pursuits that can be healing and serve as a channel for the release of emotions.

- **Healthy Lifestyle**: Eating a balanced diet, getting frequent exercise, and getting enough sleep can all help reduce stress and enhance general well-being.

Guidance and Support Groups

Significant emotional relief can be obtained by attending counseling sessions or joining support groups:

- **Support Groups**: Making connections with people going through comparable struggles helps foster a sense of camaraderie and understanding. Support groups provide a secure setting for people to exchange stories, learn new things, and get support.

- **Professional Counselling**: Counsellors and therapists may assist people with sadness and anxiety as well as help them process their feelings and create coping mechanisms. Counseling can take place in a group or individual context.

CBT stands for cognitive behavioral therapy.

Alopecia Areata's psychological impacts can be effectively managed with Cognitive Behavioural Therapy (CBT):

- **Identifying Negative Thoughts**: Cognitive Behavioural Therapy (CBT) assists people in identifying and refuting negative ideas and perceptions about hair loss.

- **Behavioural approaches**: People can create better-coping strategies and habits by using behavioural approaches.

- **Building Resilience**: CBT helps people become more resilient by assisting them in adopting a more optimistic and grounded view of life.

Developing Confidence and Self-Esteem

Increasing confidence and self-worth is essential for those with alopecia areata.

- **Self-Acceptance**: Developing self-esteem requires embracing and accepting oneself, no matter how one looks.

- **Positive Affirmations**: Concentrating on one's own accomplishments and strengths while repeating positive affirmations might help one feel more confident.

- **Looks Options**: Experimenting with various hairstyles, wigs, caps, and scarves can boost one's self-esteem and sense of comfort when it comes to looks.

Support from Family and Society

The help of friends and family is priceless:

- **Open Communication**: Fostering candid and open dialogue with loved ones about emotions and experiences can improve bonds and offer emotional support.

Participation in Support Groups: Attending support groups can help family members have a better understanding of the condition and teach them how to support others effectively.

- **Educating Others**: Clearing up confusion and creating a supportive environment can be achieved by assisting friends and family in understanding Alopecia Areata.

Issues with Children and Adolescents

Alopecia Areata in children and adolescents presents particular difficulties:

- **Parental Support**: Parents are essential in helping their children feel supported emotionally, developing a healthy self-image, and standing up for them in public and at school.

- **School Involvement**: Creating a supportive atmosphere with the help of school personnel can make kids feel more at ease and accepted.

- **Peer Relationships**: Promoting social interaction and assisting kids in forging close bonds with their peers might help kids feel less alone.

Overcoming Social Stigma

The effects of social stigma on those with Alopecia Areata can be profound:

- **Education and Awareness**: Spreading knowledge about Alopecia Areata within a community can aid in lowering stigma and fostering compassion.

- **Self-Advocacy**: People can be empowered and the effects of stigmatization can be lessened by being encouraged to speak up for themselves and educate others about their condition.

- **Positive Role Models**: Sharing the experiences of those who have effectively dealt with alopecia areata might inspire and lessen feelings of guilt.

Meditation and Mindfulness

Practices in mindfulness and meditation can reduce stress and enhance emotional health:

- **Mindfulness Techniques**: Being attentive and giving your whole attention to the present moment can help you feel less anxious and better control your emotions.

- **Meditation Practices**: Consistent meditation can improve general mental health by fostering calm and lowering stress. Particularly helpful techniques include progressive muscular relaxation, guided imagery, and deep breathing.

Extended Psychological Support

To effectively manage the persistent issues associated with Alopecia Areata, long-term psychological care is necessary.

Regular Counselling: Attending counseling sessions on a regular basis might help people stay supported and overcome new obstacles as they come up.

- **Adaptive Coping Strategies**: People can preserve emotional equilibrium and resilience by gradually building a repertoire of adaptable coping techniques.

Maintaining Support Networks: Maintaining emotional and psychological support over time requires consistent engagement with personal and professional support networks.

Alopecia Areata can have a major emotional and psychological impact, but people can effectively manage these issues with the correct coping mechanisms, support networks, and medical attention. Developing resilience and preserving mental health mostly involves developing one's sense of self-worth, getting help, and engaging in mindfulness exercises. This all-encompassing strategy guarantees that people with alopecia areata can live happy, self-assured lives in spite of their disease.

CHAPTER 8

WAY OF LIFE AND DAY-TO-DAY ADMINISTRATION

the following comprehensive guide addresses all of the topics you mentioned:

Tricks and Advice for Hair Care

Alopecia areata hair care calls for very delicate handling. Make use of gentle shampoos and conditioners, ideally ones made for delicate scalps. Avoid using too much heat styling or harsh chemicals as these can exacerbate the damage to delicate hair. To avoid damage, use wide-toothed combs or brushes made for sensitive hair. Trim your hair on a regular basis to keep it looking nice and to lighten the strain on weakening follicles.

Selecting Hairpieces and Wigs

The material, style, and comfort of wigs and hairpieces should all be taken into account. Human hair wigs give a more realistic appearance but need more upkeep than synthetic wigs, which are more costly and require more care. To avoid irritating your scalp, go for alternatives that are breathable and lightweight. To determine the finest fit and style that complements your tastes and way of life, speak with a wig specialist.

Scalp Upkeep and Care

Keeping the scalp healthy is essential to controlling alopecia areata. To maintain a clean and hydrated scalp, use mild cleansers and moisturizers. In order to stop additional irritation and damage to the hair follicles, refrain from plucking or scratching the scalp. Include scalp massages in your regimen to encourage hair development and circulation.

Cosmetics and Techniques for Camouflage

Areas of hair loss can be disguised with cosmetics to give the impression of fuller hair. Select products made especially to conceal thinning or bald spots. Try out a variety of applications, including sprays, powders, and hair fibers, to see which works best for you. For a finish that looks natural, blend the products in flawlessly with your natural hair.

Protecting the Scalp from the Sun

It's critical to shield your scalp from the sun, particularly if you have bald or thinning patches. When you are outside, cover up with a scarf or cap made of UV-resistant material. To protect sensitive skin from sunburn and other harm, apply sunscreen to the parts of the scalp that are exposed. Always reapply sunscreen, especially after spending a lot of time in the sun.

Exercise and Health

Regular physical exercise improves general health and well-being, which includes hair health. Select enjoyable activities that you can easily fit into your daily schedule. For people with alopecia areata, low-impact activities like yoga, swimming, or walking may be very beneficial. To help you achieve your fitness objectives, maintain a balanced diet and stay hydrated.

Nutritional Factors

A nutritious and well-balanced diet is a major factor in encouraging good hair development. Incorporate foods like fruits, vegetables, lean proteins, and whole grains that are high in vitamins, minerals, and proteins. Take into account supplements such as omega-3 fatty acids or biotin, but before beginning any new supplement regimen, speak with a medical expert. Avoid drastic limitations or crash diets since they might have a detrimental effect on the health of your hair.

Handling Anxiety and Stress

Alopecia areata sufferers may experience worsening hair loss as a result of stress and anxiety. Engage in stress-relieving activities like yoga, mindfulness, deep breathing, or meditation. Take part in enjoyable and relaxing activities, such as hobbies, quality time with loved ones, or relaxing music listening. If you're finding it difficult to manage your stress or anxiety, get expert assistance.

Regular Health Examinations

For the purpose of keeping an eye on your general health and treating any underlying issues that might be linked to hair loss, routine medical checkups are crucial. Make routine appointments to talk about your alopecia areata management strategy with your dermatologist or healthcare professional. Inform them of any changes in your health or any worries you may have about your symptoms or treatment.

Remaining Up to Date and Informed

Seek reliable information sources, including medical publications, advocacy groups, and healthcare specialists, to stay informed about alopecia areata. Join online forums or support groups to meet people going through similar things and exchange advice and experiences. Keep yourself informed about new breakthroughs in research and treatment options so that you can make the best decisions for your care.

You may effectively manage alopecia areata and preserve the best possible condition for your scalp and hair by including these methods in your daily regimen and way of life.

CHAPTER 9

TESTIMONIALS AND TRUE STORIES

Individual Accounts of Diagnosis

Personal narratives from people who have been diagnosed with Alopecia Areata can add a personal element to the understanding of the illness. These narratives frequently describe the emotional rollercoaster of experiencing first symptoms, being confused, going to the doctor, and then getting a diagnosis. They provide empathy and relatability to people on comparable journeys by shedding light on the anxieties, uncertainties, and concerns that surface along this process.

Traditional Treatment Experiences

For many years, topical immunotherapy, corticosteroid injections, and topical corticosteroids have been the standard therapies for Alopecia Areata. Testimonials from individuals can shed light on the effectiveness, drawbacks, and difficulties related to certain therapies. Learning about people's experiences with conventional therapy enables others to set realistic goals, comprehend possible consequences, and decide on their own course of treatment.

Emerging Therapies Success

Many Alopecia Areata patients now have hope thanks to novel medications like JAK inhibitors. Telling others about these treatments' successes might motivate and inform them about the new options available for treating the illness. These accounts, which describe the increase in hair regrowth, the effect on the quality of life, and any difficulties encountered during the course of therapy, frequently illustrate the journey from skepticism to hope.

Recovery and Adjustment Techniques

Emotional fortitude is just as important as physical control in managing Alopecia Areata. Narratives from personal experience about coping mechanisms and adaptation tactics offer significant perspectives on how people manage obstacles like low self-worth, societal attitudes, and psychological health. These accounts could contain strategies, tactics, and mental adjustments that have enabled people to accept their individuality and prosper in spite of their illness.

Inspiring Tales of Recovery

Stories of recovery highlight the tenacity of people who have surmounted major obstacles brought on by alopecia areata. These stories frequently feature turning points in the protagonist's development, acceptance, and self-awareness. Inspirational stories demonstrate that healing is not just physical but also emotional and spiritual, giving others going through similar difficulties hope, inspiration, and a sense of empowerment.

Perspectives from Children and Parents

Alopecia Areata can have distinct effects on kids and their families. It can be uplifting and educational to hear from kids about their experiences coping with the illness, from feeling different to embracing their individuality. In a similar vein, parents who describe their experiences raising a child with alopecia areata provide valuable perspectives on emotional support, advocacy, and building resilience in the family.

Surmounting Social Obstacles

For people with alopecia areata, social obstacles like stigma, prejudice, and misinformation are frequent. Narratives from personal experiences overcoming these obstacles highlight the significance of consciousness, learning, and self-defense. Additionally, they demonstrate the vital role that communities, advocacy groups, and support groups play in fostering inclusive and encouraging settings.

Perspectives from Long-Term Survivors

Those who have lived with Alopecia Areata for a long time have important life lessons to share. Their tales frequently demonstrate adaptability, resiliency, and a profound awareness of self-acceptance. These realizations highlight the value of patience, self-care, and overall well-being and can provide direction, knowledge, and perspective to those who are either newly diagnosed or having difficulty managing their condition over the long term.

Takeaways and Suggestions

Lastly, it can be quite beneficial to share knowledge gained and helpful suggestions from individual experiences with Alopecia Areata. These pearls of wisdom, which may include hair style methods, skincare regimens, stress management strategies, or insights from personal growth experiences, can help people dealing with comparable difficulties. Real-life experience-based advice is more relevant and actionable because it is relatable and honest.

CHAPTER 10

RESEARCH AND FUTURE PATHS

Recent Trends in Research

Currently, research on alopecia areata is concentrated on a few major trends. Understanding the intricate interactions between genetics, the immune system, and environmental variables in the onset and progression of alopecia areata is one important field of study. Additionally, researchers are investigating cutting-edge therapeutic modalities like immunotherapy and regenerative medicine. Personalized medicine and the application of AI to enhance diagnosis and treatment results are also receiving more attention.

Genetic Research Breakthroughs

The hereditary mechanisms underlying alopecia areata have been clarified by recent advances in genetic research. Research has revealed particular genes and genetic variations linked to the illness, offering important new understandings of its etiology. These discoveries may open the door to individualized treatment plans based on a patient's genetic profile and targeted treatments.

New Developments in Immunotherapy

One promising method of treating alopecia areata is immunotherapy. The creation of biologics that target immunological pathways involved in the illness process is one example of this field's breakthroughs. The goals of these treatments are to promote hair growth and regulate the immune system. The optimization of immunotherapy regimens and the discovery of biomarkers to forecast treatment response are the main areas of ongoing study.

Regenerative Medicine Advances

Using regenerative medicine to stimulate the body's natural healing processes, alopecia areata may be effectively treated. To promote hair follicle regeneration, researchers are looking into methods like stem cell therapy, platelet-rich plasma (PRP) injections, and tissue engineering. For those suffering from alopecia areata, these developments provide hope for more potent and durable therapy alternatives.

Personalised Medical Interventions

Personalized medicine techniques are transforming the management of alopecia areata by customizing therapy regimens to each patient's specific needs, taking into account their immune system, genetic composition, and degree of the condition. Better results and increased patient satisfaction result from this tailored strategy, which minimizes adverse effects while optimizing therapy efficacy.

Future Treatment Options

New therapeutic approaches that target particular biological pathways linked to hair loss may be used to treat alopecia areata in the future. These could include combination medicines that target several elements of the disease process, small molecule inhibitors, and gene editing approaches. Trials in humans are being conducted to assess the effectiveness and safety of these possible remedies.

Artificial Intelligence's Function

Research and clinical practice related to alopecia areata are seeing an increasing amount of involvement from artificial intelligence (AI). Large datasets are analyzed, patterns are found, and disease outcomes are predicted using AI algorithms. Additionally, this technology is being used to create individualized care plans, treatment algorithms, and diagnostic tools, improving the accuracy and efficacy of alopecia areata therapy.

Participation of Patients in Research

Research involving patients is essential to improving our knowledge of alopecia areata and creating efficient therapies. In order to help researchers create more patient-centered studies, patients can provide insightful information about their experiences, preferences, and treatment outcomes. Involving patients as collaborators in research fosters openness, confidence, and cooperation among the scientific community.

Research Ethics: A Consideration

Informed permission, patient privacy and confidentiality, and maintaining integrity and transparency in study design and reporting are all ethical considerations in alopecia areata research. To guarantee that research findings benefit a variety of patient populations and reduce inequities in access to care, researchers must also take equity, diversity, and inclusion into account.

The Prospects for Alopecia Areata Treatment

The treatment of alopecia areata has a bright future thanks to continuing improvements in patient involvement, technology, and research. Anticipate increasingly individualized and successful treatments that are catered to the specific requirements of each patient, driven by advancements in regenerative medicine, immunotherapy, genetic research, and artificial intelligence integration into clinical practice. Guided by ethical principles and a dedication to improving patient outcomes and quality of life, patient participation in research will remain crucial in determining the future landscape of alopecia areata therapy.